The Ketogenic Diet
Strategy

Successful Tips & Tricks To Power Through

Christopher J. Lewis

TABLE OF CONTENTS

INTRODUCTION

Thank you for purchasing the book "Ketogenic Diet Strategy: Tips And Tricks To Power Through".

In this book not just do I help you comprehend what the Ketogenic eating routine is about additionally share a few formulas for the different dinners you will devour as the day progressed. As the Ketogenic diet comprises of expending a lot of fats, proteins and utilizations a low measure of carbs, it works thinks about whether you have been attempting your best to accomplish that awesome body you have dependably wished to accomplish.

In any case, do recollect, while diets work in a basic and compelling way, it is all up to you. That is, everything relies on upon how you keep up the equalization and eat sound as well as tries to enjoy somewhat physical movement no less than three to four times each week. On the off chance that you don't lead an inactive life or your work does not include a lot of physical action, screen the admission of calories every day. On the off chance that you lead an existence which is substantial in physical movement, you should as needs be change the proportion of fat to protein to carbs appropriately. According to the Keto diet, your every day eating routine ought to incorporate a higher measure of fat, a moderate measure of protein and a low rate of carbs. While a few people assert that eating methodologies are not the most ideal route forward to getting in shape, it is simply because they attempted and fizzled. The explanation behind them coming up short is not the eating regimen but rather in fact it is on the grounds that they don't start the eating regimen on the right note or can't keep up the parity in what they eat or drink and consequently the eating routine they ought to have been on transforms into a fiasco for them!

On the off chance that you eat solid and simply eat the measure of nourishment as endorsed, there will be no halting you in effectively keeping up the Keto diet. You won't just feel lighter additionally glad!

KETOGENIC DIET
WHAT'S IT ALL ABOUT?

Before we start an eating routine it is constantly best to first comprehend what the eating regimen is about. In this part, I will clarify what Ketosis is and how tailing this eating routine could help you in your weight reduction objective.

Ketones exist in each body and are little parts of fat which are created by the liver when the body's nourishment admission is low. Ketosis is the procedure which triggers a caution of sorts to the body cells to smolder the fat delivered or the ketones in an auspicious way. At the end of the day, when your eating routine is less of carbs, the glycogen levels in your body fall and you enter the ketosis stage. When this happens, the ketones keep the proteins put away in the muscles from being utilized and rather use vitality from all the fat put away in your body.

Ketosis is an ordinary metabolic procedure that happens in your body and it is vital that you adhere to the administration and abstain from enjoying that "only one" trick dinner. On the off chance that you do avoid a specific part of the administration to enjoy a trick feast, you will lose all the advancement you have earned. It will likewise take your body a couple days before ketosis starts once more in your body. You ought to guarantee that your tricks are zero!

In normal circumstances, the body utilizes glucose as the principle type of vitality which permits the body to work. Glucose is acquired from carbs which we expend as dull sustenance things and also things which contain sugar. A large portion of the normal nourishment things which are high in carbs are bread, pasta and so on which the body then separates into sugar. This sugar is either utilized by the body or is put away in our muscles and is called glucose.

Some individuals take after the Ketogenic eat less additionally prevalently known as the Low Carb Diet. The point of this eating routine as I had disclosed above is to copy fat and utilize the same for vitality as opposed to depending on carbs.

As we learned over that ketosis is the point at which the body utilizes the fat put away as a part of the body to make vitality as opposed to depending vigorously on carbs. The Ketogenic diet or the low carb diet makes the metabolic state in the body which then guides in weight reduction.

In the Ketogenic diet, around 75% of the eating regimen includes fats and fat based nourishment things. Around 20% compensates for the protein utilization in the eating regimen leaving around 5% of the caloric admission to be gotten from carbs.

A study which was distributed in the American Journal of clinical sustenance in 2008 watched that a gathering of hefty persons taking after the Keto diet for around 4 weeks lost a normal of 12lbs. The members in this concentrate additionally specified that they could expend less calories without feeling as ravenous as they would ordinarily feel because of a diminished measure of carb admission.

Since our bodies are accustomed to changing over the carbs into glucose, when we restrict the measure of carbs being expended, our body enters ketosis. Our liver begins separating fat cells into unsaturated fats which is then spent as vitality.

Advantages Of The Ketogenic Diet

1. The Ketogenic diet works since we diminish or constrain the calories we devour once a day, along these lines your body blazes more vitality than it gets because of the caloric deficiency. One of the best preferences of the Ketogenic eating routine is its capacity to help the body control hunger successfully when contrasted with different eating methodologies.

2. The Ketogenic diet controls the glucose and lessens the expansion in insulin delivered every day. When we devour a great deal of carbs, for example, breads or other boring sustenance items, the glucose level in our blood increments. The insulin then scatters the glucose which results in those craving throbs you feel routinely. Since the Keto diet requires low carb consumption, our glucose levels are kept up and diminish the yearning throbs.

3. The Keto diet permits you to eat sustenance which satisfies your yearning and keeps you full for more hours. On the off chance that you are taking after the Keto slim down legitimately, you will find that every day you will expend the vast majority of your calories from dinners high in fat and protein. These suppers

keep your appetite under control as well as guarantee you appreciate what you eat.

The Ketogenic eating routine is not a prevailing fashion eating regimen nor is it something new, in fact this eating routine has been around for quite a long time and is picking up unmistakable quality at this point. At the point when the Keto eating routine is actualized accurately, it is to a great degree successful for enhancing one's metabolic wellbeing.

HOW TO GET STARTED WITH KETO

Getting Started With The Ketogenic Diet

For an eating regimen to be fruitful, one needs to dependably take after an eating routine arrangement. Whether it's a cutting edge eat less carbs, a 7-day challenge or a lone juices diet, there is dependably a period table of nourishments that is put down and took after. Likely in light of the fact that once you begin an eating regimen, you'll be excessively eager, making it impossible to arrange at every progression, so it's ideal on the off chance that you arrange ahead of time!

Through the whole span of the eating routine, the body gets re-prepared to take a gander at all the sustenance's entering your body. On consistent days before beginning the eating regimen, your body is taught to assault the carbs settled in your stomach first and final then proceed onward to the fats. Be that as it may, in the Ketogenic diet, if your carb consumption has been extraordinarily minimized, the body is in all probability going to assault what it can see most in the body-which is the majority of the solid fats. Since they are the more advantageous of the fats, the body can retain it a mess quicker and less demanding, and is thusly wrecked no sweat. Ketones are put energetically to haul out whatever undesirable fats are available in your body and change over them into new fuel for the body to keep running on.

Clear your House of the considerable number of Goodies

If you are going to give it your everything, you should start with this tip. Get out your concealed stash of treats stacked with sugar or things which are substantial in carbs. The kitchen drawer, your bedside drawer, the ice chest, packs or your own particular pantry. We've all been there! Get everything out. Give away the sustenance things you need to keep away from to a man in more prominent need of everything.

Read and Re-read the Guidelines

Don't simply wrap up this book and hurl it aside. Make a note of all the sustenance things you are intended to keep away from, and the ones you are permitted to eat.

Set a Date for yourself

Help yourself by beginning this amid a non-Christmas season or a period when you have practically no social responsibilities.

Tell Everybody!

Go ahead; tell the entire world in the event that you need to, once you do, you know there is no retreating. Along these lines individuals will likewise recognize what you won't eat on the off chance that you do get welcomed to a last moment get together that you completely need to go to.

Plan Ahead

Now, when I say arrangement, I mean arrangement your suppers, plan for a day in the week where you go looking for foodstuffs you require. When you have a rundown for goods, stick to it!

Get a Keto diet Buddy

Get your closest companion, family, kin, and partner from work, anyone why should willing hold your hand and bolster you to likewise share in this eating regimen. Incase no one needs to go along with you, there are a lot of online Keto diet gatherings where you can motivate conversing with individuals who have achieved great wellbeing from doing the Keto diet. That ought to rouse you facilitate.

Make a List

Of the considerable number of things you can eat and can't gobble and put it up in spots you visit a ton. To begin with, clear out your fridge first then perhaps your workspace and other kitchen cabinets at home. That will make it a considerable measure simpler for you to avoid enjoying unfortunate pigging out sessions.

Journal It!

Get yourself a diary; make it a propensity once a day to record how you felt in the wake of having a specific nourishment thing. That way, you can likewise monitor how your body has responded to the great and the awful. This will likewise help you track the measure of fats, proteins and above all the amount of carbs you have expended in a day.

It is not Just a Diet

When you start dispensing with grains, sugar and so forth from your day by day diet, you won't just advantage short-term, however on a long haul premise too. Try not to do this in the event that you think it is simply one more in vogue diet. Do it for yourself and your wellbeing.

Keep it Simple

Your nourishment does not need to speak to some lavish lodging menu. Keep your feast arranges straightforward, formulas can be speedy and simple to make.

List Of Food And Beverages To Avoid

The sustenance things recorded beneath are what drive up your insulin levels in the body.

1. Sugar and whatever other sweetened sustenance things. Make certain to peruse names and comprehend the different names for sugar said on the bundling.

2. Grain and grain products like bread, pasta.

3. Corn and any corn items. Corn can be found in everything as corn syrup or as an additive, so read the name painstakingly before you simply ahead and buy an item.

4. Potatoes and sweet potatoes

5. Canned soups/stews and ready to eat bundled sustenance things

6. Processed foods

7. Beans like lima beans, pinto beans, lentils are high in starch

8. Rice

9. High carb beverages

   - Beers

   - Dessert wines

   - Non-diet soda

   - Juices from vegetables and fruits

   - Milk, contains lactose which is likewise a sort of sugar. However drain items, for example, yogurt and cheddar have a lower measure of lactose as the microorganisms which are utilized to age the milk gobbles up all the lactose amid the maturation procedure of the cheddar.

Once your body gets used to the sound changes and changes to a more advantageous method for eating, it will understand that it doesn't need to function as hard as before with regards to separating sustenance in the framework. This implies your liver isn't under as much stretch as it was beforehand. Since your framework is no more obstructed with unfortunate handled nourishment things or sustenance containing an abnormal state of sugar and its by items, inside weeks of starting the eating routine, you will wind up feeling much lighter and you won't have an excessive number of sustenance longings also.

Before you start the Keto Diet, you should guarantee that you have had a storeroom intercession. On the off chance that you can't motivate yourself to do it, ask a companion or a nearby relative or your life partner to bail you out. On the off chance that you pick the sack of treats over a modest bunch of nuts or sunflower seeds, or cook a cluster of chips as opposed to setting up your cuts of meat, then you require wash room mediation immediately!

Getting executioner advantages out of the Ketogenic eating regimen will require you to show order and duty in adhering to eating the right sort of sustenance.

Make the procedure less demanding on you by taking a stock of your kitchen and storeroom stockpiling ranges. Look through the foods grown from the ground that you have in stock, make note of your supply of Omega-3 unsaturated fat alongside other essential sources of energy which your body receives.

Eat To Your Content With The Keto Diet

Once you've made the decision to beginning the Ketogenic Diet, you've guaranteed yourself a superior and a more advantageous way of life. Presently it just stays for you to start an eating routine arrangement and stick to it!

Given beneath is likely how you can arrange your days further:

- Go through the sustenance list that you can eat.

- Break it down into fats, carbs and proteins.

- Now, plan a dinner to-feast menu for regular of the eating routine

- You can start by including the sort of menu arranged out for him or her

- Start your breakfast with meat rubbed in flavors and herbs alongside a touch of olive oil to roll it. It's obvious that you are cheerful comfortable start of this eating regimen!

- For lunch you can have a much heavier supper plates of mixed greens in spread, pork slashes in garlic cream all joined by servings of mixed greens in either farm dressing or whatever other low carb dressing.

- The thought behind this eating regimen is to stack your dinners with protein consolidated with high fats, furthermore picking low carb veggies to round it off with. The thought is not to starve you, but rather to eat enough inside as far as possible.

KETO DIET RECIPES

Recipe 1: Scrambled Eggs With Onions And Nuts

Serves: 2

Nutritional Values

Calories	199
Calories from Fat	23%
Carbs	6g

Scrambled eggs are a great way to start your day. Here is a yummy recipe for your famished stomachs.

Ingredients Required:

3 eggs

1 cup sliced onions

½ cup tomatoes

1 tablespoon olive oil

1 tablespoon pine nuts

Salt and pepper to taste

Method:

In a frying pan, pour in the olive oil and add in the onions and cook till golden brown. Add the tomatoes and fry for 5 minutes. Remove the mixture from flame and set it aside.

In a bowl, whisk the eggs well, add salt and pepper according to your taste. Next add in the onion and tomatoes into the egg mixture.

Now cook the egg mixture on low flame and stir continuously until it is scrambled well. Add in the pine nuts. Remove from heat and serve.

Recipe 2: Bacon and Eggs

Serves: 3

Nutritional Values

Calories	378
Calories from Fat	30%
Carbs	35.6g

This is a classic breakfast dish which is super quick and easy to make and is an absolute treat.

Ingredients Required:

100 grams bacon rashers

8 egg whites

Pepper and salt to taste

1 onion

1 tablespoon olive oil

Method:

In a frying pan, pour in the olive oil. Cook the bacon on a medium flame. Chop the onions finely and add it in the frying pan. Keep stirring until it turns brown. When the onions and bacon are cooked, add in the egg whites and scramble it altogether. Sprinkle with pepper and salt and serve with lettuce.

Recipe 3: Banana Pancakes

Serves: 4

Nutritional Values

Calories	520
Calories from Fat	26%
Carbs	55g

These fluffy pancakes are really a great inclusion in your Keto diet.

Ingredients Required:

1 cup banana

1 tablespoon coconut oil

2 tablespoons butter

Handful of chopped almonds

1 egg

Method:

In a bowl, mash the bananas well. Add in the butter and grated almonds and blend it well. In a frying pan, heat the coconut oil on medium heat. Place the pancake mixture in the frying pan and cook it well. Flip it over to cook the other side.

Recipe 4: The Keto Casserole

Serves: 4

Nutritional Values

Calories	560
Calories from Fat	37%
Carbs	60g

Casseroles are a great breakfast option that can be stored for a few days. This breakfast casserole recipe is something that your whole family can enjoy. This recipe includes sweet potato and although too much of it should not be consumed, it provides the amount required for your daily carb intake when you are on the Keto diet.

Ingredients Required:

1 small onion

1 sweet potato

Pork sausage

1 cup spinach

2 tablespoons olive oil

5 eggs

½ cup coconut milk

Dash of nutmeg

Salt and pepper to taste

Method:

Preheat the oven to 400 degrees Fahrenheit. Add in the olive oil, salt and pepper and roast them in oven for 15 minutes. Cut and sauté your onions in olive oil till the onions are caramelized.

Next cook the sausage on medium heat. In a separate bowl, whisk the eggs, almond milk, nutmeg, salt, and pepper. Blend it well.

In a baking dish, assemble the browned sausage at the bottom followed by the caramelized onions and roasted potatoes. Top it with the spinach. Next pour in the egg and coconut mixture to cover all the ingredients.

Bake at 350 degrees Fahrenheit for 20-30 minutes.

Recipe 5: Nutty Salmon

Serves: 3-4

Nutritional Values

Calories	371.6
Calories from Fat	32%
Carbs	7g

If you are in the mood for something with a little crunch and a nutty texture, this dish is your best bet. Fry this in a pan with some bacon fat or clarified butter and you are in for a treat!

Ingredients Required

5-6 salmon fillets; 2.5-3 inches thick

1.5 cups mixed sesame seeds (white and black); you could also use snapper or any other white fish

Salt and pepper

Clarified butter, bacon fat or coconut oil for frying

Method

Wash the fillets and pat them dry. Sprinkle salt and freshly crushed black pepper on both sides of the fillets.

In a plate spread out the sesame seeds, place one side of the salmon on the sesame seeds, do the same for the other side. Melt whatever oil/fat you are using for frying the salmon.

Keep the flame on medium, since you do not want the seeds to burn and the fish to be raw. Gently place down the fish in the pan, cooking each side for 4-5 minutes. Once both sides are cooked, remove it gently and let it rest before serving.

Note: This dish pairs beautifully with a baby spinach and rocket leaves/arugula salad.

Recipe 6: Chicken With Veggies

Serves: 3-4

Nutritional Values

Calories	570
Calories from Fat	18%
Carbs	78g

Here is a skillet-cooked mix of chicken and veggies with a lively taste.

Ingredients Required:

1 small chicken

5 onions

1 cup mushrooms

2 teaspoons vinegar

1 teaspoon olive oil

1 cup chicken stock

1 bay leaf

2 sprigs thyme

2 oz bacon

¼ cup butter

2 tablespoons parsley

1 teaspoon tomato paste

Method:

Cut the chicken into small pieces. Marinate the chicken with vinegar, thyme and bay leaf for 30 minutes. In a skillet, fry the bacon till it is well cooked. After it is cooked set it aside. In the skillet over medium heat, sauté the mushrooms in a little butter for 5 minutes. Remove from flame and set it aside.

Next add in little more butter to sauté the onion till it is golden brown. Set it aside. Drain the marinated chicken pieces and keep the remaining marinade in the side. Melt all the remaining butter and throw in the chicken pieces and cook well.

Add the remaining marinade, chicken stock and add in the bacon. Next add in the onions and mushrooms. To this add in the tomato paste and cook for 30 minutes.

Recipe 7: Stir-Fried Asparagus And Beef

Serves: 2

Nutritional Values

Calories	350
Calories from Fat	21%
Carbs	70g

Asparagus, beef, parsley and other healthy ingredients combine to make this delicious main course.

Ingredients Required:

1 onion

1 bunch green asparagus

2 bell peppers (you can use either red bell peppers or a mix of all three bell pepper colors)

1 garlic clove

1 ½ cups roughly chopped bite size beef pieces

1 tablespoon ginger

Parsley

Coconut oil

Salt and pepper to taste

Method:

Finely chop the onion, red peppers, asparagus, and ginger. Stir-fry the vegetables one by one and set aside. In a wok, add in some coconut oil to stir-fry the beef strips and cook over high heat.

Next add in the garlic and onion., the asparagus and bell peppers and stir fry for another few minutes. Finally season it with the ginger, salt and pepper.

Garnish it with parsley.

Recipe 8: Keto Chocolate Cake

Serves - 4

Nutritional Values

Calories	550
Calories from Fat	25%
Carbs	66g

Nothing says dessert like a good chocolate cake. Here is a fabulous Ketogenic diet cake recipe to try.

Ingredients Required:

1/3 cup coconut flour

½ cup dark chocolate

5 whole eggs

3 separated eggs

¼ cup coconut oil

1 teaspoon vanilla extract

Method:

In a bowl, add in the 3 egg white and beat it till you stiff peaks. Using the double boiler technique melt the dark chocolate. In another bowl, add in the 5 eggs, the 3 yolks and keep mixing. To this add the coconut flour little by little.

Next add in the coconut oil and melted chocolate and keep stirring in one direction. Fold in the egg whites into the mixture. Add in the vanilla extract. Pre-heat your oven to 180 degrees Celsius. Grease the cake tin and line it with baking paper. Pour the mixture into the cake tin.

Bake in the oven for 40 minutes at 180 degrees Celsius. Allow the cake to cool before serving.

Recipe 9: Passion Fruit And Mango Sorbet

Serves - 2

Nutritional Values

Calories	176
Calories from Fat	5%
Carbs	40g

Indulge yourself in this cool and refreshing sorbet recipe.

Ingredients Required:

2 passion fruits

1 mango

1 egg white, beaten until stiff peaks have formed

Method:

In a bowl, beat the egg whites till you have stiff peaks. Using a blender, blend the mango and passion fruit together till you have a creamy texture. Fold the egg whites into the mango mixture. Pour it into a freezer proof container and freeze for 6 hours or until it has set.

While serving cut into slices and top it with mango or passion fruit slices.

Recipe 10: Salmon With Mushroom

Serves - 2

Nutritional Values

Calories	367
Calories from Fat	18%
Carbs	75g

Salmons coupled with creamy mushrooms make one scrumptious meal.

Ingredients Required:

4 pieces king salmon steaks

1 cup mushrooms

1 tablespoon olive oil

½ cup chicken stock

1 tablespoon garlic

3 tablespoons butter

½ tablespoon thyme leaves

2 tablespoons shallots

1 tablespoon lemon juice

Salt and pepper to taste

Parsley leaves

Method:

Sprinkle olive oil on the salmon fillets. Season it with salt and pepper. In a heavy pan, sauté the mushrooms and keep it aside.

Grill the fish till it is well cooked. In the pan add the shallots and garlic and add in the chicken stock. Keep heating till the liquid is half, add in the thyme.

In another pan, reheat the mushrooms with butter. Remove the salmon from your grill and top it with the mixture.

Garnish with parsley and lemons while serving.

TIPS TO POWER THROUGH

Stay Hydrated

This is seen as a simple choice, however is hard to take after. We consistently get so involved in our day-day encounter that we disregard to hydrate sufficiently. I endorse super hydrating your structure by drinking 32 oz of water inside the essential hour of waking and another 32-48 oz of water before twelve.

Practice Intermittent Fasting

This is a standout amongst the best ways to deal with get into and keep up ketosis since you are lessening calories and not eating up protein or carbs. It is a brilliant thought to go low-carb for no not exactly several days prior to starting this with a particular deciding objective to avoid a hypoglycemic scene.

Eat up Enough Good Salts

We are told in our overall population that it is fundamental to reduce our sodium utilization. Various individuals in our overall population fight with a high sodium/potassium extent. This is a result of the way that when we are on a higher sugar diet, we regularly have higher insulin levels.

When we are on a low sugar, ketogenic diet, we have lower insulin levels and in this way our kidneys release more sodium which can provoke a lower sodium/potassium extent and a more essential necessity for sodium in the eating regimen.

Get Regular Exercise

Needless to say, just eating the right way but not exercising is not going to help you power through this eating regimen. Even if you don't get enough time, park your car a little further from your workplace and walk or take the stairs. At the end of the day you have got to ensure you are moving and not just eating all day.

Make an effort not to Eat Too Much Protein

Various people doing a Ketogenic diet eat up an overabundance of protein. In case you eat up over the top protein than your body will change the amino acids into glucose through a biochemical method called gluconeogenesis

Pick Carbs Wisely

We in general understand that a ketogenic eating routine is a low-carb mastermind anyway I endorse using supplement rich sugar sources, for instance, non-dull veggies and little measures of low-glycemic regular items like lemon, lime etc..

Hold Stress Down

Unending nervousness will shut down your ability to be and stay in ketosis. If you are encountering an extreme a great time, than keeping up ketosis may not be the right target. This doesn't mean you should begin carb stacking, however rather reset your target to simply keep centered lower carb, quieting diet.

Improve Your Sleep

If you are resting inadequately, you will raise stress hormones and cause glucose deregulatory issues. Make sure to set yourself up to go to rest at a conventional time and rest in an absolutely diminish room. I propose snoozing at least 7 hours consistently depending on your uneasiness levels (more extend means you require more rest) and the aggregate you feel as though you need to feel awesome and judiciously caution for the span of the day.

CONCLUSION

I trust this book could help you comprehend the Ketogenic Diet, and has even propelled you enough to begin it. While this may not give you the precise intricacies of the eating routine, it will give you an expansive thought of the whole eating regimen and how one ought to approach it.

While you do experience this eating regimen it is vital to recollect a couple of basic tenets to make the procedure a ton simpler for you. A decent practice administration supplements the Ketogenic Diet, so tie up your shoelaces and head down to the rec center or for a run. Pair it up with a couple home activities or weights and you will promptly see the distinction.

Through the course of the eating regimen, it is likewise imperative to have the capacity to attempt and make however many dinners as could reasonably be expected, independent from anyone else. This will guarantee the validness of the suppers in your eating routine and in addition let you realize what precisely goes into the sustenance you are expending.

In particular, before you start this eating regimen or some other, it is crucial to counsel a specialist or a dietician with the goal that they will have the capacity to guide you all the while. For whatever length of time that you don't push your points of confinement with this eating regimen and eat right, you ought to see 'another you' soon!

Good Luck!

FROM THE AUTHOR

If you found this book useful, please take the time to share your thoughts and post a review on Amazon.

It'd be greatly appreciated!

Thank You!

www.ingramcontent.com/pod-product-compliance
Lightning Source LLC
Chambersburg PA
CBHW062029280526
45787CB00005B/2256